I0427851

How to obtain Kissable Lips

Volume 1

How to obtain Kissable Lips-Volume 1 | 2014

Table of Contents

Dedication's Page

This book is dedicated to every man or woman that wishes to obtain kissable lips for 2014

This book is also dedicated to my family and friends. They have loved me more than I have loved myself

This book is also dedicated to my betrothed if and when I ever find him.

Introduction

Every man and woman would always like to know how to obtain soft and smooth kissable lips. If they follow these simple routines, they could make their lips more inviting to the human eye as well as much more attractive.

Exfoliation

Everyone needs to remember to exfoliate their lips as often as they can. This will remove any dead skin cells that may be present on your lips.

A person should use either their chosen lip serum or lip creams from their favorite provider. A person can also use home made remedies such as a small amount of sugar, water and vinegar.

You should exfoliate your lips at bedtime.

Lip Polishing at Bedtime after Exfoliation

A man or woman should always apply some petroleum jelly or Vaseline at bedtime. They could apply some lip balm or common chap stick immediately after the exfoliation process.

If you apply a chap stick or lip balm equipped with some SPF, you could also avoid any sun damage that could occur while you are out.

Relaxation of the lip muscles

Lips can get some tension inside them and this could make your mouth feel and look tightened and tense. If your lips look clenched all of the time, your lips could look less kissable to everyone. Obviously, you do not want this!

A person can make their lips more relaxed simply by allowing their lips to move slightly apart. By leaving just a small sliver so that air may move through them, this technique will allow your lips to appear more fuller and well relaxed.

Framing your lip shape

A man or woman needs to establish and maintain lip symmetry. This is more important than the fullness of your lips. Always remember that lip symmetry is the beacon of universal attractiveness.

For any female, they should always remember to wax any hair from their upper lip. Especially, if they have pale complexion and dark hair. The waxing will make your lips actually "pop" and give your lips essential contrast between your lips and your skin.

A woman should also use a lip liner so that it will smooth out any imperfections that could be present before applying a tinted lip gloss or their favorite lip shade which correlates to their skin tone.

For the males, stubble can be a very big problem! Always remember that extra long kissing could irritate your partner's facial complexion.

Every guy knows that facial hair can hide slight imperfections that they may not be comfortable with.

Stubble can present a common denominator between a youthful appearance and that it signals masculinity.

If a man smokes, eventually, they can obtain "smoker's lines" on their upper lips. The "smoker's lines" will make your lips look less attractive to another person.

Making eye contact and smiling seductively always helps lip attractiveness

If a person smiles seductively from across the dinner table or from across the room, this will draw attention from your partner.

If you look like you're happy and curl the corners of your lips upwards, this will always show off your kissable lips.

__You should establish a morning and evening beauty regimen for your lips on a daily basis__

When you brush your teeth before bedtime, always remember to rub a moist towel across your lips when you are finished. This technique will remove any dead skin cells that may be present on your lips.

If you actually brush your lips with a dry toothbrush, this routine will exfoliate your lips also. This in turn can make your lips soft, supply and absolutely kissable.

You should always try to add a little bit of Vaseline on your lips before bedtime. Try not to use a lot of chap stick because it can dehydrate your lips after a while. This is what you want to avoid, if at all possible.

Always remember to keep the Vaseline on all night!

The use of moist towels

In the morning while getting ready for the day, always try to rub a moist towel on your lips. This method will in fact hydrate your lips and remove excess skin cells that could be present on your lips from the night before.

Lip colorization and liners for your lips

A woman should always try to use a lip liner that correlates with their chosen tinted lip gloss or their favorite lip shade. The lip liner will prevent the lip color from bleeding into your skin.

You should try to apply your lip color evenly and smoothly as possible.

Providing shine and lip gloss to your daily make-up routines

A woman should always remember that the appearance of greasy lips is very unattractive indeed! They should always put a medium drop of lip gloss on their upper and lower lips. You should always try and even it out as well.

Always remember to keep your mouth open for about twenty seconds before your close your mouth.

A man or woman should always remember to hydrate their bodies with a lot of H2O

If you have cracked and dry lips, this is a definite sign of dehydration. When you hydrate your body, it definitely shows. A man or woman would notice that their cracked lips, sunken eye sockets and bony fingers look much better.

The End

How to obtain Kissable Lips-Volume 1 is a self-help guide to assist any man or woman who would like to achieve attractive kissable lips for their partners. If you follow these steps, you should definitely notice a difference in your lips appearance.

Misty Lynn Wesley has a very diversified career portfolio in the medical, legal and fashion industries. Her love of fashion, beauty and genetics were her inspirations in writing this self-help book to obtain kissable lips.